Make Your Own Herbal Teas At Home

By Gabrielle Lilly,

LMT, MA, Certified Herbalist

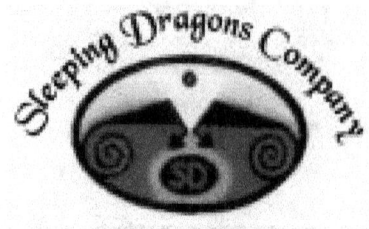

Sleeping Dragons Company

Be Excellent!

Make Your Own Herbal Teas At Home
By Gabrielle Lilly
ISBN-13:
978-1546846567

ISBN-10:
1546846565
FunFast Productions

This book includes some
basic information about making herbal tea at
home.
IT DOES NOT CONTAIN ANY MEDICAL
ADVICE, and is not meant to replace necessary
medical treatments of any kind. It also does not
contain all the information there is to know on
this topic, or anywhere close to it.

This information is a broad and brief overview of
the topic of tea and a basic introduction to a
simple process which is easy to do at home.
Mostly, it is a collection of recipes and general
information about many popular herbs that are
used for medicinal teas.
 It is my hope that interested readers like you
will take this information as a starting point and
be inspired to learn more about the topic.

There are infinite variations in methodology and ingredients possible and this little book can only introduce a basic understanding which it is then up to you to build upon. I have included several popular recipes and some information about several individual herbs commonly used to make healing herbal teas, which you can use to formulate and make tea for yourself and for your family that may help many common ailments.

Again, these are not meant to take the place of proper medical treatment, and they are not medical advice! Please seek proper medical attention for any serious ailment or disease. Also, these are only a brief introduction, and you are encouraged to experiment and expand on this knowledge to get the best benefits from it for yourself and your loved ones.

Remember, we all are in this together...so be excellent!

About the Author:
Gabrielle Lilly has been practicing the Art and Science of Herbology among family and friends for more than 25 years. She is a NM State Licensed Massage Therapist and Nationally Certified Bodyworker and considers herself a novice Certified Herbalist, and Aromatherapist.

At the time of writing this, there are no national or state recognized licensure programs for herbology. Gabrielle did receive a certificate of completion for an extensive home-study course in the Art and Science of Herbology, which was written by Master Herbalist Rosemary Gladstar, in 2000. She has also participated in numerous weekend seminars and various specialty healing weekend workshops, including Reiki, Aromatherapy, Neuromuscular Therapy and Trigger Point Therapy.

Gabrielle considers learning a life-long endeavor. She is an Artist, Singer, Songwriter, Practical Healer, Trickster Clown, and Alternative Builder. Her current focus includes Music, Unity, Positive Alignment, and Balancing Masculine and Feminine Energy. She runs a thriving eBay store that specializes in Natural Creativity Supplies.

You can find her store on eBay at http://stores.ebay.com/Sleeping-Dragons-Company, or find her on Facebook, YouTube, Twitter, Instagram, LinkedIn, Reddit, Tumblr, and other social networks as Gabrielle Angel Dee Lilly, or Angel Lilly.

www.sleepingdragonsco.com
www.deluxaromas.com
www.funfastco.com
www.absoluteacres.com
www.angellilly.com

"A cup of tea would restore my normality."
— Douglas Adams, The Hitchhiker's Guide To The Galaxy Screenplay

"There are those who love to get dirty and fix things. They drink coffee at dawn, beer after work. And those who stay clean, just appreciate things. At breakfast they have milk and juice at night. There are those who do both, they drink tea."
— Gary Snyder

"When tea becomes ritual, it takes its place at the heart of our ability to see greatness in small things. Where is beauty to be found? In great things that, like everything else, are doomed to die, or in small things that aspire to nothing, yet know how to set a jewel of infinity in a single moment?"
— Muriel Barbery, The Elegance of the Hedgehog

"There is something in the nature of tea that leads us into a world of quiet contemplation of life."
— Lin Yutang, *The Importance of Living*

"If you are cold, tea will warm you;
if you are too heated, it will cool you;
If you are depressed, it will cheer you;
If you are excited, it will calm you."
— William Ewart Gladstone

A Brief Overview of "Tea"

Making tea is easy and fun!

The tradition of tea-making goes back many centuries. There are probably infinite variations on methods and recipes.

Tea leaves in the strictest traditional sense come from a specific plant (chamellia sinensis). This tea comes in white, green or black (roasted). Oolong tea is made from the same type of mature leaves, which are fermented first and then roasted. White tea is usually immature chamellia sinensis leaves, though sometimes other plants are used. Gunpowder tea is again the same type of plant, but the whole leaves are rolled into individual balls and then dried so they look like little pellets. These leaves unfold when they are steeped in hot water.

There are many slight variations in botanical varieties and processing techniques. Geologic locations, fluctuating weather conditions, and storage conditions also affect the flavor, therapeutic properties, appearance, and price of teas and other herbs.

Another factor that affects the flavor and chemistry is the quality and temperature of the water it is brewed in. Of course, how long the tea is brewed also effects the flavor. It's better to err on the side of lower water temperature. The delicate leaves of white and green teas require below boiling water temperatures between 170 and 185 degrees Fahrenheit. Too high of a temperature will cook the leaves and ruin their delicate flavors. Tea leaves like Oolong should be brewed at temperatures between 180 and 190 degrees Fahrenheit. Heartier black tea and most herbal teas brew best at a full boil temperatures 208 and 212 degrees Fahrenheit.

Many teas are flavored by the addition of herbs and sometimes essential oils, such as peppermint or bergamot. Jasmine or honeysuckle flowers are a popular addition to many traditional teas. Cut fresh or dry leaves of peppermint, spearmint, lavender flowers, and rose petals also blend quite well with traditional tea leaves. There are also many herbal combinations that are prepared the same way as tea leaves, and though these are not actually "tea" in the strict, traditional sense.

Any beverage prepared with water and leaves of chamellia sinensis or any other plant bits is commonly called "tea" in American culture. These can be leaves, flowers, roots, barks, and berries. Usually, preference is given to those with a pleasing flavor and or aroma, though sometimes pleasing flavor is sacrificed somewhat for therapeutic benefit. I think a really good tea should be healthy, and taste wonderful too!

It is worth noting, that leaves and flowers are generally more delicate than roots and barks and most berries. The tougher your herbal material is, the harder it will be to extract flavor and other therapeutic properties from it. Roots and barks may need to be broken up into smaller pieces and will need to be steeped in hot or simmering water for longer than more delicate leaves and flowers. They may even need to be simmered over low heat for awhile (5-15 minutes).

Technically speaking, in the herbal medicine world, if you steep your herbs for longer than about 15 minutes then the resulting liquid is called an "infusion" and if you simmer them for any length of time the result is called a "decoction". Most of us would simply call it "tea", unless it tasted really bad. If you do simmer your herbs, be sure to keep them covered and keep the heat as low as possible.

Herbal Chai tea blends are a common example of a popular tea drink that is best simmered very briefly, and then steeped for a good while for a fuller flavor. Chamellia sinensis, or botanical tea leaves contain some caffeine, which is another reason they should not be boiled or simmered for any substantial length of time. Over-steeping or overheating them can burn delicate tea leaves and flowers, and cause excess acidity in tea. This can cause bitterness, and even give the person who drinks the tea a nasty headache.

The study of tea growing, trading, making, and drinking is a rich enough subject to keep many a doctoral student busy for years. If you are interested, I suggest you do an on-line search or spend a day at your local library digging into it. Better yet, start your own tea party tradition. Invite a new friend or group of friends over to share a cup of tea.

The basics of tea-making are as simple as pouring a cup of very hot water over a spoonful of tea leaves or herbs and waiting 5-15 minutes until the water extracts some of the properties of the tea or herbs, or until the water is 'infused' with properties of the tea. Even though you will find many documented rituals and sometimes complex traditional methods for preparing tea, there is nothing wrong with simply pouring a cup of hot water over herbs and enjoying the end result. Don't be limited by other traditions, if you want to make your own tea ritual, feel free to!

Some people prefer to sweeten their tea with sugar, honey, agave syrup, or stevia, and some like to add a splash of milk to their tea, particularly black tea or herbal tea blends that contain black tea. Of course, all that is a matter of personal preference, and I encourage you to experiment to find what you like best.

A good rule of thumb for making herbal tea is to start with about one teaspoon of dry chopped herbs or leaves per six ounces of hot water, though there can be great variation in this amount, according to taste. Personally, I like about twice that amount for most teas; most of the time. Usually the tea leaves or herbs are removed or strained out before optional sweetening and drinking, although that is not always necessary. Some herbs are fine to leave in the water. They will usually sink to the bottom eventually, much like coffee grounds will if you make "cowboy coffee".

If you use a teapot to steep your herbs in, then you can use some type of tea-ball or strainer, or you can leave the herbs or tea loose in the teapot to steep. It is much easier to clean your teapot later if you contain your leaves in a tea-ball, muslin bag, or something else made for steeping tea. I prefer to use a muslin draw-string bag I have for this purpose whenever I am making more than one cup of tea, as it is reusable after a quick rinse.

How To Make Sun Tea:

Instead of hot or boiled water, you can use the sun's heat to make tea. You can drink the tea while it is hot from the sun, or you can chill it and make iced tea. If you are making iced tea, be sure to sweeten it while it is still warm if you prefer additional sweetener. Of course, you can always sweeten it cold, but once the tea cools down it will be harder to dissolve most sweeteners in it. Obviously if you use herbs, such as Stevia or Licorice, to sweeten the tea or if you prefer unsweetened tea, then this is not an issue.

One of my favorite things in the summer is iced herbal Sun Tea. This process captures healing properties from the sun as it infuses water with your tea and/or herbs. I start with a 4"x6" clean muslin drawstring bag, about a cup of herbal tea or mixed herbs, and a clear glass jar.

I fill the muslin tea-bag about two-thirds to three-fourths of the way full with my favorite herbs or herbal tea blend. I prefer to use muslin bags because they are re-useable after a quick rinse.

I place my home-made giant tea-bag into a gallon-sized glass jar. I often pour a cup or two of purified hot water over it at this point just to get everything started. This is not necessary, unless you want or need to speed things up. I have a wonderful electric teapot sized water heater which I got as a gift from my little brother, and which heats a cup or two of water to a boil in practically no time at all! I would not have thought I would like it, but I love it because I can make tea in minutes now. Since I got it, I have added this step to making Sun Tea because it is so easy and it does get the tea "juices" going.

I fill the jar up with pure, cold water and cover it with clear plastic wrap. I usually secure the plastic 'lid' with a large rubber band. I like to meditate over it at this point or give a quick expression of gratitude or blessing. There is increasing evidence that our thoughts have a great impact on our material world and that positive thoughts have the ability to affect the quality of water more quickly and dramatically than most of us might think. I encourage you to look up Dr. Masaru Emoto's work if you are interested in the potential effects of prayer on water.

I place my tightly covered jar outside in direct sunlight. I live in a very sunny climate so getting hot enough is never a problem. If you live in a colder climate you might want to make a solar oven or solar collection area for Sun Tea if you really want to 'get serious' about it. The idea is that the sun heats up the water hot enough to infuse the water with flavors and healing properties of the herbs, while also infusing healing properties from the sun. I have a special smooth piece of dark granite stone outside in the sun where I brew my Sun Tea, but anywhere that gets direct sunlight for most of the day, preferably at least 5-7 hours or so, should be fine.

I often leave my sun-tea out overnight to soak up reflective moonlight, and bring it in to refrigerate in the morning. If you use a little stevia leaf in your herbal tea blend it will already be naturally sweet! Make sure you keep your sun tea refrigerated, and drink it all within 2-3 days, as it may start to go bad after that. Adding sugar or honey can increase the shelf-life a little.

A Note About Strainers:

Most people use a strainer of some kind to make tea. There are various types of tea balls, metal strainer spoons, bamboo strainers, and muslin cloth bags. Just about any strainer will work just fine, though some styles work better for certain types of teas or herbal mixtures. Experiment and find what works best for you. Remember to consider the type of teas you make, the particle size, or cut, of the herbs or teas you use, and the container you make it in, as well as your personal style of course!

A Few of My Favorite Popular Herbal Tea Blends:

The following are brief descriptions and ingredient lists for some popular herbal tea blends. The exact amount of each herb to use is up to you. Usually they can be modified to suit your taste or to match what you have available to you in your herb cabinet. As you become more familiar with herbs you will probably find there are some flavors you prefer over others. These ingredient lists are generally listed from most to least, as is customary in all ingredient lists. Usually they are mixed up by the quart or by the pound, and then brewed by the single cup or by the tea-pot-full (or jar-full for sun-tea). You can make delicious iced-tea with just about any hot tea. Simply make your tea extra strong, sweeten it if you want it sweet, let it cool a bit, then chill it over ice and/or in the fridge.

Oatstraw Dream Tea:
Ingredients-Chamomile, oatstraw, linden flower, scullcap, catnip, lemon verbena, fennel, wild lettuce, nutmeg, and calendula.

Relaxing and Calming, this blend of flowers, herbs, and spices, this tea presents a complex medley of flavors to ease your mind and body. Chamomile and linden flowers induce serenity and help melt your stress away with the help of oatstraw, catnip, and skullcap. This tea has a fruity and fresh flavor which is further complemented by the floral bouquet of chamomile and calendula. Sweet dreams!

Chai Tea:
Ingredients commonly include- Cinnamon, ginger, cardamom, black tea, allspice, cloves, and black pepper.

Increasingly part of the popular culture, Chai Tea has been blended for centuries in Southern Asia. True to the variability inherent to making tea, each family recipe subtly unique. There are many variations of Chai, but most contain at least cinnamon, ginger, cardamom, cloves, and black pepper. Since I like caffeine, Chai just isn't Chai to me without a hearty helping of black tea. I prefer it like most Americans; served with cream and sugar. Chai is amazing both hot and iced; perfect for summer and winter treats!

For a Caffeine Free Chai Tea, simply remove the black tea.

Chamomile-Mint Tea:
Ingredients-Chamomile and peppermint leaves.

An herbal tea that is perfect for after a meal, Chamomile-Mint combines the digestive properties of peppermint with the settling relaxation of chamomile.

An aromatic and blissful tea, this blend also opens up the airways, focuses on the stomach, and eases away stress and distraction. This unique combination can slow down the mind while invigorating the digestion process. Drink this one on the couch and let the day slip away!

Cold & Flu Brew:
Ingredients- Peppermint, elder flower, rosehips, ginger, anise seed, thyme, yarrow, and calendula.

This is a helpful blend to help ease symptoms of almost any common cold or flu. Its' benefits come from a variety of tastes that energize the body and keep it functioning at peak performance.

Ginger and anise seed stimulate your immune system, while peppermint and yarrow work at removing causes of illness. Elderflower flushes out your system, and rosehips top you up with fantastic vitamin C. This light refreshing cup packs a protective punch that is safe for nursing moms and most children too!

I like to add elderberry and wild cherry bark tincture to this mixture if I am really battling something serious.

Get Smarter Tea:
Ingredients-Peppermint, gota kola, ginkgo, lemon grass, ho shou wu, eleuthero root, licorice, damiana, and calendula.

This tea is formulated to stimulate your mind and improve your concentration and memory.

These herbs work together to create a "cornucopia of tastes" and an abundance of health benefits. While gotu kola, eleuthero root, and ginkgo focus your mental abilities, Ho Shou Wu, peppermint, damiana, and calendula arouse the body's energy. With lemongrass and licorice to harmonize the herb medley, this herbal tea is a complete tonic, mind and body.

Hibiscus Mint Tea:
Ingredients-Hibiscus, peppermint and stevia.

Red petals and green leaves are blended together to create this simple but magnificent herbal tea. Hibiscus Mint is made of only three ingredients, but these powerhouses of flavor can carry their weight! The lightness and freshness of mint produces a feeling of freedom, while the floral notes of hibiscus blossoms are soothing and relaxing. Sip it slowly or drink it quickly. Hot and soothing or iced and refreshing; this tea feels fantastic!

Licorice Mint Tea:
Ingredients- Peppermint, licorice root and cloves.

Any peppermint infusion carries an effervescent airiness about it, a weightless sparkle of energy and light. Licorice Mint herbal tea is no exception. Described as a fresh earthy taste with a lasting sweetness, licorice makes up the other half of this taste adventure. A third flavor comes with the gentle spark of cloves, a faint shadow of smouldering warmth. Revel in three unique taste experiences which blend into their own fantastic flavor!

Moroccan Mint Tea:
Ingredients- Peppermint and yerba mate.

Mix about half and half yerba mate with peppermint and you have one of the best every day drinks around! This popular combination makes an excellent hot or iced tea, and is both stimulating and soothing, all at the same time!

Life-Loving Tea:
Ingredients- Licorice, yerba santa, dandelion root, yellow dock, nettles, and rosemary.

It's too easy in life to forget about our health, yet hardly anything is more missed when it is absent! This blend is a healing blend of traditional herbs used for the internal cleansing and rejuvenation of your body. Naturally sweetened with licorice and yerba santa, this tea also combines dandelion root, yellow dock, nettles, and rosemary into a pale green infusion that is loaded with goodness!

Mama Mia Tea:
Ingredients- Raspberry leaf, nettle, spearmint, ginger, oatstraw, rose petals, lemon balm, and chamomile.
An herbal tea designed just for the expecting woman, this blend is especially formulated to supply a wealth of health benefits towards the end of pregnancy. Nettle soothes the body's aches, while oatstraw elevates your overall mood. Raspberry leaf is known to ease labor, and chamomile and lemon balm contribute to calmness of mind and body. Spearmint and ginger, the ultimate body tonics, maintain your health as you await your bundle of joy!

Wiccan Woman's Tea:
Ingredients- Raspberry leaf, vitex, nettles, linden flower, lemon verbena, lemon peel, cinnamon, roses, and stevia.

This blend of herbs combines flowers, fruits, and leaves to achieve a balanced tonic for health and happiness. Rich in iron, this profusion of ingredients includes raspberry leaf, vitex, nettles, linden flower, and cinnamon. Deliciously balanced with fruity and floral notes of luscious lemon and radiant rose, and a final lingering sweet note of stevia. Magically delicious hot or iced!

Yogini Tea:
Ingredients-Cinnamon, cardamom, ginger, black pepper.

This traditional herbal blend brings together the familiar spices associated with Chai and Garam masala. It is formulated to sooth and aid digestion and balance the body's energies. With a permeating warmth in every cup, this delicious "flavor parade" is also equally wonderful over ice as it is piping hot! I enjoy this one with a little milk and honey, similar to my Chai tea.

Some Common Herbal Ingredients Used In Tea:

It is important to use clean, pure water to start. You may want to spend a little extra time purifying, or even praying, or focusing positive energy over your water to improve the quality of your tea.

The quality of your tea leaves or herbs is important as well. Use the freshest herbs you can for the best tasting tea! The following is a brief, introductory summary and overview of information about just a few of the many common herbs that are used to make tea or as ingredients in herbal tea blends. This information is for educational purposes only and is NOT meant as medical advice whatsoever.

It is my hope that you will be inspired to learn more about herbs and natural healing if you so choose. This information is meant only as in introduction and is does not tell anywhere near all there is to know about any of the plants listed. This is also only an introductory list, and is not even close to a list of all the popular herbs used in herbal tea blends. I encourage you to learn more, to experiment, and to share your experiences!

Alfalfa: *Medicago sativa*: a blood purifier; reduces and prevents symptoms caused by arthritis, bursitis, and gout; lowers cholesterol. Alfalfa contains eight essential digestive enzymes and eight essential amino acids of protein, and a high chlorophyll content. It is an extremely rich source of Beta-Carotene, Minerals, Trace elements, and vitamins A,B-1, B-6, B-12, C, D, E, K, Biotin, Folic Acid, Niacin and Pantothenic Acid. Mineras are Calcium, copper, Iron, Magnesium, Phosphorus, Potassium and Zinc.

Catnip: Cats like to nip this plant, as it seems to affect them as an aphrodisiac and a euphoric. Catnip doesn't cause the same behavior in humans, but it is particularly beneficial because of its excellent sedative, digestive and nutritional properties. Like many botanicals, Catnip has many excellent nutritional properties, and the leaf of Catnip is highly valued in herbal medicine.

The primary chemical constituents of Catnip include essential oils (carvacrol, citronellal, geraniol, nepetol, nepetelactone, pulegone, thymol), iridoids and tannins. It also contains iron, selenium, potassium, manganese, chromium and other nutrients. Catnip has soothing and relaxing effects on the digestive system, relieving diarrhea, flatulence, indigestion and upset stomach.

Catnip contains antispasmodic properties that are said to be useful for treating abdominal and menstrual cramping, as well as chronic coughing. Thought to be excellent for reducing fevers, Catnip's antibiotic and astringent properties are considered beneficial for treating colds and bronchial infections. Catnip's sedative qualities have also been used to alleviate sleeplessness, insomnia and headaches.

Chamomile flowers: Chamomile makes a tasty beverage by itself and is also a wonderful addition to many blends. Chamomile tea is often given to infants and children to help calm them or to help manage symptoms of a cold. It is considered one of the safest herbs and has long been revered for its ability to calm and relax the entire body. Its natural soothing properties make it valuable for supporting healthy nervous system function. Chamomile also soothes the gastrointestinal (GI) tract, and is often used to help ease a nervous stomach.

Contraindications:
Those who suffer from allergies to members of the daisy family (ragweed) should consult a doctor or allergist before using Chamomile. Chamomile contains natural blood thinners (coumarins) and should not be taken by those using the prescription drug Coumadin or other blood thinners. Because Chamomile is a uterine stimulant, pregnant women should discuss its use with their physicians before using it. Chamomile may also cause drowsiness.

Cinnamon Bark: In ancient times, Cinnamon was added to food to prevent spoiling, and it was used in Egypt for embalming. During the Bubonic Plague, sponges were soaked in Cinnamon and Cloves and placed in sick rooms, and it has also been burned as an incense. During the explorations of the fifteenth and sixteenth centuries, Cinnamon was the most sought-after spice.   The fragrance of Cinnamon is pleasant; stimulates the senses; yet it calms the nerves, and it is reputed to attract customers to a place of business.

Most Americans consider Cinnamon a simple flavoring, but in traditional Chinese medicine, it's one of the oldest remedies, prescribed for everything from diarrhea and chills to influenza and parasitic worms. It is closely related to Cinnamonum Cassia, which is primarily sold as cinnamon in the US and contains many of the same components, but the bark and oils from Cinnamon have a sweeter flavor which is considered superior.

Cinnamon has a broad range of historical uses in different cultures, including the treatment of diarrhea, rheumatism and certain menstrual disorders. Traditionally, the bark was believed best for the torso, the twigs for the fingers and toes. Recent research has highlighted hypoglycemic properties, useful in diabetes.

Cinnamon may help relieve nausea and vomiting, and, because of its mild astringency, it can be particularly useful in infantile diarrhea. The cinnamaldehyde component can lower blood pressure and help to decrease spasms by increasing peripheral blood flow. The essential oil of this herb is a potent antibacterial, antifungal and uterine stimulant.

Contraindications:
Pregnant women or those allergic to Balsam of Tolu should not use Cinnamon. Men with prostate problems, diabetics and those taking blood thinners should consult a health care provider before using Cinnamon. This product is not recommended if you have a tendency toward excessive menstrual bleeding. Taking Cinnamon and antibiotics together may make the antibiotic not work for you. Increased heart rate (pulse), feeling dizzy, shortness of breath and redness of the face may occur if you take too much Cinnamon.

Chrysanthemum: These flowers have long been used to alleviate fever and headaches and also to disperse and remove toxins from the body. They are excellent for counteracting inflammation and are said to be effective in relieving symptoms of vertigo. They are thought to help improve vision and are used for a wide range of eye problems such as soreness, redness, night blindness and strain. The flowers are also known to purify the blood, and in Chinese Medicine, they are used as a cooling summer beverage.

Chrysanthemum is considered anti-inflammatory, antipyretic and antihypertensive. Chrysanthemum flowers have been used to relieve hypertension and vertigo; to pacify the liver; expel wind and clear eyesight.

Contraindications:
People with allergies to daisies or asters should not use Chrysanthemum, as it may produce an allergic reaction. Those who are weak or have diarrhea should not use the herb.

Corn Silk: was used traditionally as a mild diuretic and is said to be helpful for irritation of the urinary system and also as a urinary demulcent, combined with other herbs, for cystitis, urethritis and prostatitis. Corn Silk has been used for renal problems in children, and Chinese research indicates that Corn Silk may reduce hypertension and blood clotting time.

Derived from the dried silky tassels found inside the husks of corn, Corn Silk acts as a diuretic and has been used to reduce the formation of sediments in the kidneys, relieve inflammation caused by urinary tract problems and help reduce water retention in the body. It is said to help alleviate conditions of painful swelling and a wide range of genito-urinary complaints.

Cornsilk has also been used in conditions of high uric acid, such as gout and some types of arthritis, and it may also alleviate prostate disorders, including difficulty in the beginning of urination. Corn Silk contains mucilage and has been used to soothe irritation in the kidneys and bladder, often caused by burning and painful urination. It is also thought to relieve irritation of the bladder and urinary tract by coating the membranes that line the urinary system walls.

Corn Silk contains iron, silica, potassium, vitamins B, C and K and also contains moderate amounts of zinc, calcium, magnesium and phosphorus. Its key constituents are considered to be maizenic acid, fixed oil, resin and mucilage.

Chicory Root: This common root is often used as a caffeine-free substitute for coffee, has also been used medicinally in the treatment of gout, dyspepsia and jaundice. In contrast to coffee, Chicory Root is a natural sedative and is also used as a diuretic and mild laxative. The roots are commonly dried and ground to make a caffeine-free coffee substitute, although the plant does have a bitter flavor. Medicinally, Chicory has been used to treat skin disorders, gout, jaundice and to reduce an enlarged liver.

Contraindications:
Pregnant and nursing women should not use Chicory Root.

Dandelion: This well-known plant is more than just a common lawn weed; it is one of the planet's most famous and useful weeds. Dandelion contains many vital nutrients, minerals and vitamins A, B, C and D. It has been used for centuries as a primary herb that purifies the blood and flushes toxins out of the body, via the liver and kidneys.

Contraindications:
Pregnant and nursing women should not use Dandelion. It is not recommended for people with gallstones or biliary tract (bile duct) obstruction without first consulting a physician. In cases of stomach ulcers, gastritis or irritable bowel, Dandelion should be used cautiously, as it may cause over production of stomach acid.

Those who are allergic to daisies or asters should not use Dandelion. Do not take Dandelion without talking to your doctor first if you are taking certain medicines used to treat infection (antibiotics such as Cipro, Tequin, Levaquin, etc., as it may lower efficacy of drug); Potassium supplements for health condition (too much may be harmful); Blood thinning medicine (Coumadin, Plavix, aspirin, etc.).

Ginger Root: Ginger is an amazing catalyst for other herbs, though it is most commonly known for its effectiveness as a digestive aid. Chinese ships carried pots of Ginger aboard when on long sea voyages to prevent scurvy and sea sickness, and a Chinese folk remedy recommends rubbing the cut root of the plant on the scalp to stop hair loss.

Ginger Root has also been used for centuries in Chinese herbal medicine for the positive effects it has on the body. Ginger's sweet taste has made it a popular herb, and it is found today in ginger ale, breads, candies and tonics. By increasing the production of digestive fluids Ginger can enhance the effectiveness of herbal combinations.

Ginger may help to relieve indigestion, gas pains, diarrhea and stomach cramping. The primary known constituents of Ginger Root include gingerols, zingibain, bisabolenel, oleoresins, starch, essential oil (zingiberene, zingiberole, camphene, cineol, borneol), mucilage and protein. Ginger Root is also used to treat nausea related to both motion sickness and morning sickness and is said to be the most effective herb for curbing motion sickness, without causing drowsiness.

Ginger's anti-inflammatory properties are thought to help relieve pain and reduce inflammation associated with arthritis, rheumatism and muscle spasms. Ginger's therapeutic properties are believed to effectively stimulate circulation of the blood, removing toxins from the body, cleansing the bowels and kidneys, and nourishing the skin.

Other uses for Ginger Root include the treatment of asthma, bronchitis and other respiratory problems by loosening and expelling phlegm from the lungs. Ginger Root may also be used to help break fevers by warming the body and increasing perspiration.

Contraindications:
People taking blood thinners (Coumadin, aspirin, etc.) should avoid Ginger, and the herb should be avoided for two weeks prior to elective surgery. Pregnant women who use Ginger for morning sickness should not take large amounts (many times the recommended dose) nor use it for prolonged periods without consulting a physician. Ginger increases bile production and should not be used by people with gallstones or gallbladder disease unless supervised by a doctor.

Hibiscus: This attractive flower has been used to ease indigestion, relieve colds and respiratory trouble, as well as an aid to good circulation. Hibiscus is commonly made as a tea to ease stomach trouble and is also a natural source of vitamin C.

Hibiscus grows in tropical areas throughout the world, and has been used not just as an ornament, but also as a medicine for centuries. The part of this plant used medicinally is the flower, and it was used by the Chinese to treat dandruff and stimulate hair growth. Hibiscus has also been used to treat hemorrhoids and wounds.

Hibiscus has a mild flavor and has many culinary uses, and the flower is made into a tea in numerous cultures throughout the world. Research has shown that Hibiscus Flower may have antibacterial properties. It is considered a mild laxative, and it contains vitamin C and malic acid. Hibiscus has also been shown to relax the uterus and reduce blood pressure. The herb has also been used for indigestion and loss of appetite, as well as for colds, respiratory problems and circulation disorders.

Honeysuckle: The flowers of this plant have been used for centuries in Chinese medicine for treating inflammation, fever and infection. The herb has also shown promise in combating certain malignant diseases and is already highly regarded as an antibiotic that combats infection both internally and externally. Honeysuckle has also been used as a laxative, diuretic and blood purifier. Honeysuckle has been used medicinally in China for generations, where it is employed in Traditional Chinese Medicine to clear heat and toxins from the body, but it has only recently been adopted by Western herbalists.

Honeysuckle is a natural source of salicylic acid, the compound from which aspirin is made, and can thus be used in cases of headache, joint pain and fevers. Honeysuckle has been used as a gargle for sore throats and mouth ulcers, and it may also be used as a mild laxative, diuretic and diaphoretic. Topically, Honeysuckle has been used to ease the pain of sunburn and reduce the itching of poison ivy and other rashes.

Contraindications:
Pregnant and nursing women should not use Honeysuckle.

Lemon Balm: This herb is not only tasty, it is also said to have the ability to heal wounds, ease indigestion, relieve menstrual cramps, fight cold sores (herpes simplex), relax nerves, soothe minor wounds and insect stings, help prevent sleeplessness and even repel mosquitoes. This is a safe herb for children, and it tastes very good. Lemon Balm had been used for centuries, having early references found in Roman writings and was sacred in the temple of Diana.

Lemon Balm is an excellent carminative herb that may relieve spasms in the digestive tract, and is used in cases of flatulent dyspepsia. It has been described by some herbalists as being restorative to the nervous system, similar in some ways to Oats. It may be used in conditions of migraine that are associated with tension, neuralgia, anxiety induced palpitations and/or insomnia. Lemon Balm is also believed to have a tonic effect on the heart and circulatory system, causing mild vasodilation of the peripheral vessels, thus acting to lower blood pressure. It can be used in feverish conditions, such as influenza.

Contraindications:
Lemon Balm is mild, gentle and safe for children. It is wise, however, not to take it concurrently with barbiturates for insomnia or anxiety, as it may increase their effects. With regard to the Essential Oil (only) of Lemon Balm, persons with glaucoma should avoid it, as animal studies show that it may raise the pressure in the eye.

Lemongrass: This common cooking herb has been used to treat internal parasites, stomach disorders, hypertension and fever. The herb has also been shown to contain antifungal and antimicrobial properties. Lemongrass is used in herbal teas and other nonalcoholic beverages, and the oil of Lemongrass is used in candy and baked goods, as well as a topical treatment for athlete's foot, ringworm and muscle soreness. Oil from lemongrass is also widely used as a fragrance in perfumes and cosmetics, such as soaps and creams.

When taken internally, Lemongrass is considered a carminative and is also believed to have antimicrobial and antifungal properties. It is also thought to act as a central nervous system depressant. Lemongrass is a specific remedy against nematodes, and the oil shows activity against some bacteria.

The herb contains five constituents that are thought to inhibit blood coagulation. Lemongrass has been used to relieve skin problems, sore throats and respiratory problems. In traditional medicine, Lemongrass is used to combat anxiety, insomnia, stomach problems, hypertension and fever.

Licorice Root: Licorice tastes great and also helps cleanse the colon, supports lung health and promotes adrenal gland function. Licorice is a common ingredient in throat-soothing herbal supplements, and its natural sweetness makes it a favorite flavor in herbal teas and many food products. Ancient cultures on every continent have used Licorice Root, included recorded use by the Egyptians in the third century B. C. The Egyptians and the Greeks also recognized the herb's benefits in treating coughs and lung disease, and it was so highly valued in ancient Egypt that even King Tutankhamen was apparently buried with a supply.

The most common medical use for Licorice Root is for treating upper respiratory ailments including coughs, hoarseness, sore throat and bronchitis. This herb is thought by some herbalists to be as effective as codeine, and possibly safer, when used as a cough suppressant. Rhizomes in Licorice have a high mucilage content which, when mixed with water or used in cough drops, sooths irritated mucous membranes. The use of Licorice also has an expectorant effect which increases the secretion of the bronchial glands.

Today, herbal preparations containing Licorice Root are used to treat stomach and intestinal ulcers, lower acid levels and coat the stomach wall with a protective gel. Rarely used alone, Licorice is a common component of many herbal teas as a mild laxative, a diuretic and a carminitive for flatulence. It has also been thought to relieve rheumatism and arthritis, regulate low blood sugar, and may be effective for Addison's disease (under the doctor's care).

The Root extract produces mild estrogenic effects and it has proven useful in treating symptoms of menopause, regulating menstruation and relieving menstrual cramps. The constituent, glycyrrhizin, is fifty times sweeter than sugar, making Licorice a widely used ingredient in the food industry. The distinctive flavor of Licorice Root makes it a popular additive to baked confections, liqueurs, ice cream and candies. It is also widely used in other medicines to mask bitter tastes and also to prevent pills from sticking together.

Licorice has also been used in poultices for treatment of dermatitis and skin infections. It helps to open the pores and is used in combination with other cleansing and healing herbs as an emollient. Ninety percent of the Licorice imported into America is used to flavor tobacco, and other uses of Licorice include cattle and horse feed.

Contraindications: Licorice is a powerful herb and should be treated with respect. Pregnant women, diabetics and those with high blood pressure should avoid this herb. People suffering from heart disease should not use Licorice unless under a physician's care. According to the German Commission E monograph, Licorice supplements are contraindicated in people with liver and kidney disorders, and thus, people with kidney disease, gallbladder disease and cirrhosis should avoid this herb. Large doses of Licorice may induce sodium retention and potassium depletion and can lead to hypertension and edema. Use of Licorice should be done under the supervision of a health care provider or qualified practitioner.

Licorice is not meant for long term use and should not be taken for more than seven days in a row. Long-term intake of products containing more than one gram of glycyrrhizin (the amount in approximately ten grams of root, which is far in excess of the daily dosage recommended by this product) is the usual amount required to cause these types of effects.

Do not take Licorice without speaking with your physician if you take the heart medication, Digoxin (Lanoxicaps®, Lanoxin®, Lanoxin Pediatric®) or prescription diuretics (which may lead to loss of potassium, which may cause fatigue, muscle cramps, headaches, swelling, increase urination, breathlessness or high blood pressure). Other possible drug interactions with any Licorice product include potentiation of anticoagulants and possible interference with hormonal therapy due to estrogenic activity of Licorice (including decreased testosterone and birth control pills).

Meadowsweet: This pleasant smelling herb is considered a mild antispasmodic and sedative. This herb is a forerunner of aspirin, as salicylic acid was first synthesized from Meadowsweet in 1835. It is gentler on the stomach than aspirin, because Meadowsweet contains natural buffering agents. Meadowsweet also helps to reduce inflammation.

The primary chemical constituents of Meadowsweet include essential oil (salicyladehyde, methylsalicylate, hyperoside), salicylic acid, spireine, gaultherine, spiraeoside, flavonoids (rutin, spiraeoside), vanillin, glycoside, mucilage, tannin, coumarins and vitamin C. The presence of aspirin-like chemicals explains Meadowsweet's action in reducing fever and relieving the pain of rheumatism in muscles and joints.

Meadowsweet is also considered an excellent digestive remedy. This herb combines well with Marshmallow and Chamomile, with which it is very soothing for a whole range of digestive problems. It protects and soothes the mucous membranes of the digestive tract, reducing excess acidity and alleviating nausea, and it can be used in the treatment of heartburn, hyperacidity, gastritis and peptic ulceration. For musculo-skeletal conditions, consider combining Meadowsweet with Black Cohosh, Willow Bark and/or Celery Seed for their anti-inflammatory effects.

The anti-inflammatory action of the salicylates in Meadowsweet makes it effective against rheumatic pain, while the tannins and mucilages appear to buffer the adverse effects of isolated salicylates which can cause gastric bleeding (excessive aspirin can cause gastric ulceration). Phenolic glycosides, such as monotropitin, yield salicylic aglycones, which contribute to the anti-inflammatory and diuretic actions.

The astringent tannins make Meadowsweet a useful remedy in the herb's treatment of diarrhea in children. Topical applications of this herb have included its use as an eyewash for conjunctivitis and sore eyes and as a compress for rheumatic joints. Oil from the buds was used in perfume, and flowers were soaked in rainwater as a complexion water. The flowers were also used as paint brushes.

Contraindications:

Those who are allergic to aspirin should not use Meadowsweet. It is not recommended for pregnant or nursing women without first consulting a physician, and children under the age of sixteen years of age with symptoms of flu, chicken pox or other types of viral infection should not use Meadowsweet, because, like aspirin, there may be a risk of developing Reye's syndrome. Do not take Meadowsweet and bloodthinning medicine together, including nonsteroidal anti-inflammatory agents; this may cause your blood to be too thin, making you bleed or bruise more easily.

Nettle: Nettle is a common wasteland 'weed' which is well known to help maintain health of the kidneys and the urinary tract. It contains high amounts of iodine, which also can make it beneficial for the thyroid gland. Nettle is also rich in vitamins A and C, iron, calcium, magnesium, potassium and chlorophyll. Nettle leaf has been shown to be anti-inflammatory by preventing the body from making inflammatory chemicals known as prostaglandins.

Nettle's root affects hormones and proteins that carry sex hormones (such as testosterone or estrogen) in the human body, which may explain why this herb has been used to help with benign prostatic hyperplasia (BPH).

As a side note, using nettle tea to water garden plants stimulates their growth and makes them more resistant to bugs. Plants growing close to Nettles tend to be stronger in their volatile oils, and when added to the compost pile, Nettles hasten breakdown. Nettle stalks are strong and can be woven to make sails or twine. When lactating animals are fed Nettles, they are said to produce more milk, and chickens produce more eggs.

Throughout Europe, Stinging Nettles are used as a spring tonic and general detoxifying remedy. In some cases of rheumatism and arthritis, this herb can be astoundingly successful. The leaves are thought to be an excellent blood purifier.

Contraindications:

Do not take Nettle if you have high blood pressure, and some people may experience mild gastrointestinal upset with the use of this herb. There are concerns that Nettle may interact with prescription medications used for diabetes, high blood pressure, sedation and inflammation; therefore, if taking these medications, please consult your physician before taking the herb.

People with fluid retention due to congestive heart failure or kidney disease should not use Nettle, nor should those who think they are coming down with flu, because the herb reduces the body's production of immune chemical interleukin-6. Because of its exceptional diuretic properties, Nettle may cause potassium loss if taken on a regular basis, and supplemental potassium or high potassium foods, such as bananas and fresh vegetables, should be included in the diet.

Oatstraw: In folk medicine this herb was used to treat nervous exhaustion, insomnia and "weakness of the nerves." A tea made from it was thought to be useful in rheumatic conditions and to treat water retention. A tincture of the green tops of Oats was also used to help with withdrawal from tobacco addiction. Additionally, Oats were often used in baths to treat insomnia and anxiety, as well as a variety of skin conditions, including burns and eczema. Highly nutritive and supportive of the nervous system, Oat Straw helps build healthy bones, skin, hair and nails.

Oat Straw is not a bona fide aphrodisiac, but it does nourish the nerves, which is thought to make tactile sensations more pleasurable. Oat Straw is one of the best remedies for "feeding" the central nervous system, especially when under stress. It is considered a specific in cases of nervous debility and exhaustion, especially when associated with depression. Oat Straw may be used with most of the other herbal nervines, both relaxant and stimulatory, to strengthen the nervous system and is also used in general debility.

Peppermint: Peppermint might be the most commonly herb used in tea and as a flavoring in other products. This herb promotes healthy digestion by soothing and comforting the stomach. Peppermint is frequently used in herbal teas and Capsules. The essential oil of this plant contains menthol, which also displays healthful powers, and is often found in throat-soothers and topical vapor rubs.

Mint is one of the most ancient of all medicinal herbs. Ancient Athenians would rub the leaves of mint on their arms to improve their endurance, and both Greeks and Romans crowned themselves with Peppermint at their feasts and adorned their tables with its sprays. They also flavored their sauces and their wines with its essence.

Peppermint is an excellent carminative, having a relaxing effect on the muscles of the digestive system, combating flatulence and stimulating bile and digestive juice flow. It is used to relieve intestinal colic, flatulent dyspepsia and associated conditions. The volatile oil in Peppermint acts as a mild anesthetic to the stomach wall, which allays feelings of nausea and the desire to vomit. This herb has long been known to relieve nausea and vomiting associated with pregnancy, as well as travel sickness.

Peppermint is also used in the treatment of ulcerative conditions of the bowel. It is a traditional treatment for fevers, colds and influenza. Where headaches are associated with indigestion, Peppermint may help. As a nervine, it eases anxiety and tension. In cases of painful menstrual periods, the herb relieves the pain and eases associated tension. Externally, it is used to relieve itching, inflammation and a variety of respiratory conditions. Peppermint oil is also a great expectorant.

Contraindications:

Pregnant and nursing women should not take Peppermint without consulting a physician. Peppermint may aggravate hiatal hernia. Those who suffer from gallbladder disorders, gallstones or blockage of the bile duct, or those who take heartburn medication (cisapride, etc.) should not take Peppermint without consulting a physician. Do not exceed dosage (many time the recommended amount), and it is also recommended to take a few days' break after two weeks' continual use. Peppermint may interfere with absorption of iron.

Red Clover: This is another common nutritional herb which has been used for centuries as a fine expectorant and an analgesic and is also a wonderful blood purifier and cleanser. Red Clover is a vitally nutritional, mineral-rich herb that is used as a great tonic for overall good health. Herbalists have long prized this herb for its traditional use as a blood purifier, expelling toxins from the bloodstream. Primary chemical constituents of Red Clover include phenolic glycosides (salicylic acid), essential oil (methyl salicylate), sitosterol, genistein, flavonoids, coumarins, cyanogenic glycosides, silica, choline and lecithin. Red Clover also contains vitamin A, C, B-complex, calcium, chromium, iron and magnesium.

Red Clover is one of the most useful remedies for children with skin problems, and because it is mild, it makes an excellent nutritional supplement for children. The expectorant and antispasmodic action give this remedy a role in the treatment of coughs and bronchitis, but especially in whooping cough, dry cough and colds.

Red Clover also increases the production of mucus and urine flow, helping relieve irritation and inflammation of the urinary tract. As a digestive aid, Red Clover stimulates the production of digestive fluids and bile. It is also said to relieve constipation and help soothe inflammation of the bowel, stomach and intestines.

Red Clover contains easily-absorbed calcium and magnesium that are thought to tone and relaxe the nervous system, relieving tension due to stress and the associated headaches, which are further relieved by the silicic acid content.

For women, Red Clover is quite special. It contains stilbene, which is believed to stimulate eostrogenic activity, thus possibly increasing fertility and reducing "hot flashes" experienced by women during menopause. It also supports the uterus with its vitamin content, and the high protein content nourishes the whole body. There is also an alkalizing effect, which is believed to improve vaginal and uterine acid/alkaline balance.

Red Raspberry: This herb has traditionally been used to support women and to promote healthy nails, bones, teeth and skin. Red Raspberry provides a wealth of nutrients including valuable minerals and vitamins B1, B3, C, D and E. Red

Raspberry leaves have been used by women for centuries as a support to the reproductive system, especially during pregnancy. When used after birthing, they can decrease uterine swelling and minimize postpartum hemorrhaging. This herb is beneficial in normalizing blood flow during menstruation and reducing painful menstrual cramps.

Red Raspberry supports the reproductive system by strengthening the tissues of the womb, increasing lactation and easing nausea caused by morning sickness. It also cleanses and prepares breasts for a pure milk supply for the nursing infant by cleansing and purifying the blood. Red Raspberry's astringent properties make it helpful in relieving diarrhea, and its antiseptic properties make it beneficial for treating sore throats and canker sores.

Contraindications:

Pregnant women should not use Raspberry until the last two months of pregnancy, and then, only under the supervision of a knowledgeable physician.

Stevia Leaf: This amazingly sweet, easy to grow herb has been used for centuries as a natural, sugar-free sweetener. Stevia Leaf has also been employed for its antibacterial properties, and is believed by some to be of help in preventing diabetes. Stevia is a safe, all-natural alternative to artificial sweeteners and refined sugar in the diet. It has been used for centuries by native Indians in Paraguay, and consumed safely in massive quantities for the past twenty years.

Stevia has also been used for alleviating bleeding gums, sore throats and cold sores due to its mild antibacterial functions. It has also been shown to inhibit the development of plaque and aid in the prevention of cavities. There have also been some claims that Stevia functions as an antidiabetic agent.

Since Stevia does not break down when it is heated, it can be used in foods that are baked or cooked; however, because it does not caramelize, brown or crystallize like sugar does, meringues and caramel may be difficult to make. The refined Stevia extracts are considered to be calorie-free and do not raise blood sugar levels. Whereas the raw herbal form of Stevia contains nearly one hundred identified phytonutrients and volatile oils, Stevia extracts contain negligible nutritive benefits.

Yarrow: Yarrow is another well-known 'wasteland herb', which has been used to stop bleeding both internally and externally for centuries. Yarrow is also thought to alleviate inflammation, reduce fevers, stimulate the appetite and encourage sweating, while expelling toxins from the body. Yarrow's astringent properties are especially helpful in stopping nosebleeds, excessive menstruation and diarrhea.

Yarrow's effects are mostly astringent. Yarrow nutritionally supports mucus membranes. It is closely related to Chamomile, both botanically and chemically. Yarrow also contains fairly high amounts of selenium, potassium, vitamins A, C, E, F and K.

Having a variety of effects on the body, Yarrow is believed to alleviate inflammation, reduce fevers, stimulate the appetite and encourage sweating, thus expelling toxins from the body. Yarrow's astringent properties are especially helpful in stopping nosebleeds, excessive menstruation and diarrhea. Yarrow is also thought to relieve muscle spasms, arthritis and indigestion.

Yarrow helps to relax peripheral blood vessels, thereby helping to improve circulation. The constituents, achilletin and achilleine, are said to aid in blood coagulation. Yarrow contains several anti-inflammatory and pain-relieving constituents, such as azulene and salicylic acid.

Contraindications:
Pregnant or nursing women should not use
Yarrow, as it is a uterine stimulant, nor should
women with heavy periods or pelvic
inflammatory disease. Continued or long-term
use of Yarrow may cause skin irritation and/or
allergic reactions. If so, discontinue its use.

Yarrow may produce photosensitivity. If using
Yarrow to treat wounds, be sure to clean the
affected area first, as the herb can stop blood
flow so quickly that it may seal in dirt or other
contaminants. People with gallstones should
avoid its use. Yarrow may cause severe allergic
skin rashes when applied topically.

Yerba Mate: Tea made from the Yerba Maté plant is the South American equivalent to coffee in the United States.   Upon drinking it, especially for the first time, it is said that one feels a remarkable inflow of strength, energy and good cheer as a direct and almost immediate result. Charles Darwin is said to have called it "the ideal stimulant". The parts of this plant used medicinally are the roasted leaves, collected when the berries are ripe.

The actions of this herb are stimulant to the central nervous system, thymoleptic, diuretic, antirheumatic, mild analgesic, tonic and depurative. The primary chemical constituents of Yerba Maté include xanthine derivatives (caffeine citronate, theobromine, theophylline), neocholerogenic acid, chlorogenic acid, beta-carotene, vitamins B and C and sulphur. The caffeine in Yerba Maté is said to stimulate the burning of fat.

Yerba Maté is sometimes combined with other remedies in the treatment of psychogenic headache, fatigue, mild nervous depression and rheumatic pains. It is believed to stimulate mental and physical energy. Its beneficial effects are mainly due to the caffeine and theobromine constituents.

Contraindications:
Pregnant or nursing women and people who suffer from insomnia should not use Yerba Maté, because of the stimulating effects of the caffeine content. The herb should not be taken with meals, since it may interfere with the absorption of nutrients, and Yerba Maté should not be used in large amounts (many times the recommended dosage), as it is a potent stimulant. Taking Maté may interfere with the actions of lithium, and this interaction might also occur with other drugs used for manic depression and mental illness (studied but not proven).

Those with liver problems should also avoid Yerba Maté. Taking Yerba Maté and the phenyl-propanolamine in certain antihistamines and diet drugs may increase blood pressure (studied but not proven). Taking Yerba Maté may interfere with the actions of several prescription drugs, and the warnings associated with caffeine apply to this plant. Those with cardiac disorders should consult a physician before taking Yerba Maté.

Glossary of Useful Terms and Definitions:

The following are some definitions of common medical terms often used when describing herbs and their healing properties. They are NOT meant to be medical advice, and they are not all the terms used in herbal medicine! They are also not all inclusive definitions. They are a brief introduction to a few common terms used in the world of herbal medicine. I encourage you to learn more if you are interested in herbal healing.

Adaptogen: An agent that causes adaptive reactions and increases resistance to stress. Adaptogens enable the body to deal with and recover from stress and disease and appear to increase SNIR (state of non-specifically increased resistance) in the human body, protecting against diverse stresses. It is usually an herb that produces suitable adjustments in the body and tends to normalize body functions. When the job is completed, they are eliminated or incorporated into the body without side effects. Adaptogens generally work by strengthening the immune system, nervous system and/or glandular system.

Alterative: Sometimes called blood cleaners, an alterative helps to gradually and favorably alter the course of an ailment or condition. An alterative helps to alter the process of nutrition and excretion and restore normal bodily function. It also acts to cleanse and stimulate the efficient removal of waste products from the system.

Analgesic: Substance that relieves pain by acting as a nervine, antiseptic, antibiotic, antispasmodic or counter irritant.

Anesthetic (local): An agent that reduces pain in an area by desensitizing the nerves. Deadens sensation.

Anodyne: Pain relieving.

Antioxidant: Compound that prevents destructive, free radical or oxidative damage to tissues or cells.

Antipyretic (also called **Febrifuge** or **Refrigerant**) **:** A substance that reduces fever and cools the body.

Anti-rheumatic: An agent that eases the discomfort of or prevents rheumatism, a condition marked by inflammation and pain in the joints and muscles.

Antiseptic: A substance that destroys bacteria and prevents infections. Also helps to prevent tissue degeneration.

Antispasmodic: A "relaxant" or "nervine" that relieves or prevents involuntary muscle contractions or "spasms," such as those occurring in epilepsy, painful menstruation or intestinal cramping.

Anxiety: A condition marked by apprehension of danger and dread, accompanied by nervous restlessness, tension, increased heart rate and shortness of breath.

Aperient: Mild laxative without purging.

Aperitive: Herbs that stimulate the appetite.

Aphrodisiac: Agent that stimulates sexual desire or potency.

Aromatic: Substance containing volatile, essential oils; often refers to those that aid digestion and relieve gas.

Astringent: A substance that contracts, tightens and binds tissues and diminishes (or arrests) internal and external secretions. Can be used to check bleeding and diarrhea.

Ayurvedic: Traditional (and ancient) system of medicine in India. (literally, "A Science of Life").

Bitter: A plant product (often aromatic) that is used as a tonic and stimulates secretions of the digestive tract and encourages appetite.

Carminative: Agent that relieves intestinal gas pain and distension by expelling gases from the stomach and bowels. Also promotes peristalsis (contraction and relaxing of bowel). Frequently improves digestion.

Cathartic: A laxative. (1) Aperient is a mild laxative that promotes evacuation of the bowels by action on alimentary canal and (2) purgative that causes copious, rapid evacuation of the bowel and generally used to treat stubborn constipation in adults.

Contraindications: Any factor that makes it unwise to pursue a certain line of treatment.

Decoction: A water extract of bark or roots prepared at a low boil for ten to twenty minutes.

Demulcent: Mucilaginous substance that acts to soothe and relieve inflammation. Softens and soothes damaged or inflamed surfaces.

Diaphoretic: Substance that produces perspiration and elimination through the skin.

Digestive: Substance that aids digestion, usually by providing enzymes from various sources.

Diuretic: Substance that increases and promotes the secretion and flow of urine.

Emetic: Substance that causes vomiting.

Emmenagogue: Substance that promotes and stimulates menstruation.

Expectorant: A substance that loosens and expels mucous secretions and phlegm from the respiratory systems and air passages. Promotes the thinning and ejection of mucus or exudates from the lungs, bronchi and trachea.

Febrifuge (also called **Antipyretic** and **Refrigerant**): Agent that lessens fever and cools the body.

Infusion: A preparation made by steeping the plant material in hot water for twenty minutes, generally making it stronger than tea.

Nervine: A substance that calms and soothes the nerves and reduces tension and anxiety. A tonic for the nervous system that eases stress, nervous disorders and nourishes the nerves.

Nutritive: Nourishes and builds body tissues.

Organic: A term commonly used to describe foods and/or that are grown without the use of synthetic chemicals, such as pesticides, herbicides, some fertilizers, and hormones.

Purgative: A substance that promotes bowel movement and increased intestinal peristalsis.

Relaxant: A substance that relaxes nerves and muscles and reduces tension, especially muscular tension.

Restorative: Substance that renews health and strength and is effective in the regaining of normal physiological activity.

Rubefacient: Herbs that, when applied to the skin, stimulate circulation in that area of normal physiological activity.

Stimulant: An herb that increases the activity or efficiency of a system or organ - acts more rapidly than a tonic herb.

Stomachic: An agent that relieves gastric disorders. It tones and gives strength to the stomach, helps digestion and improves the appetite.

Tannin: An astringent phenolic plant constituent.

Tonic: A substance that exerts a gentle strengthening effect on the body. Designed to restore enfeebled function and to promote vigor and a sense of well-being. Tonic herbs restore and strengthen individual organs and the entire system.

Uterostimulant: Substance that stimulates the uterus.

Vasoconstrictor: An agent that narrows blood vessel openings, restricting the flow of blood through them.

Vasodilator: An agent that causes relaxation of blood vessels.

Vermicide: A medicine that kills intestinal worms.

Vermifuge (also called **Anthelmintic**): A substance that destroys and expels intestinal worms.

Volatile Oil (also called **Essential Oil**): A scented plant oil used in many herbal medicines - a mixture of hydrocarbons that are less soluble in water than alcohol or fat.

Vulnerary: A substance that arrests bleeding in wounds and prevents tissue degeneration.

Disclaimer/Reminders:

This is an introduction to a vast world of knowledge, and I encourage you to learn more, experiment, and share your findings. I hope this information inspires you to learn more about natural healing and to try making herbal teas at home.

This information is presented for educational purposes only, and is NOT intended to be medical advice!

Check out the Sleeping Dragons store
on eBay at
http://stores.ebay.com/sleepingdragonscompan
y ,
on Etsy at
https://www.etsy.com/shop/sleepingdragonsco?
ref=l2-shopheader-name ,
or at www.sleepingdragonsco.com .
Thank you!

Remember, we all are one, so be excellent to yourself!